Safety and Risk in Society Series

CHEMICAL SAFETY BOARD

SAFETY AND RISK IN SOCIETY SERIES

Chemical Safety Board
Robert W. Talford (Editor)
2009. ISBN 978-1-60692-586-7

Safety and Risk in Society Series

CHEMICAL SAFETY BOARD

ROBERT W. TALFORD
EDITOR

Nova Science Publishers, Inc.
New York

Copyright © 2009 by Nova Science Publishers, Inc.

All rights reserved. No part of this book may be reproduced, stored in a retrieval system or transmitted in any form or by any means: electronic, electrostatic, magnetic, tape, mechanical photocopying, recording or otherwise without the written permission of the Publisher.

For permission to use material from this book please contact us:
Telephone 631-231-7269; Fax 631-231-8175
Web Site: http://www.novapublishers.com

NOTICE TO THE READER

The Publisher has taken reasonable care in the preparation of this book, but makes no expressed or implied warranty of any kind and assumes no responsibility for any errors or omissions. No liability is assumed for incidental or consequential damages in connection with or arising out of information contained in this book. The Publisher shall not be liable for any special, consequential, or exemplary damages resulting, in whole or in part, from the readers' use of, or reliance upon, this material.

Independent verification should be sought for any data, advice or recommendations contained in this book. In addition, no responsibility is assumed by the publisher for any injury and/or damage to persons or property arising from any methods, products, instructions, ideas or otherwise contained in this publication.

This publication is designed to provide accurate and authoritative information with regard to the subject matter covered herein. It is sold with the clear understanding that the Publisher is not engaged in rendering legal or any other professional services. If legal or any other expert assistance is required, the services of a competent person should be sought. FROM A DECLARATION OF PARTICIPANTS JOINTLY ADOPTED BY A COMMITTEE OF THE AMERICAN BAR ASSOCIATION AND A COMMITTEE OF PUBLISHERS.

LIBRARY OF CONGRESS CATALOGING-IN-PUBLICATION DATA
Available upon request
ISBN: 978-1-60692-586-7

Published by Nova Science Publishers, Inc. ✤ *New York*

CONTENTS

Preface		vii
Chapter 1	Summary of Findings	5
Chapter 2	CSB has not Fully Addressed Key Recommendations, and Problems Persist	9
Chapter 3	Inspector General Oversight is still Warranted	15
Chapter 4	Conclusions	17
Chapter 5	Recommendations for Executive Action	19
Chapter 6	Matters for Congressional Consideration	21
Chapter 7	Agency Comments and our Evaluation	23
Enclosure I	Scope and Methodology	27
Enclosure II	Slides from April 17, 2008, Briefing to Congressional Staff	29
Enclosure III	Comments from CSB	55
Index		71

PREFACE

CSB has implemented some GAO and IG recommendations related to improving its operating policies and procedures since we last reported in July 2000. However, we found that CSB has not fully addressed several critical recommendations, and problems in governance, management, and oversight persist. Specifically, CSB has not fully responded to key recommendations related to investigating more accidents that meet statutory requirements triggering CSB's responsibility to investigate, improving the quality of its accident data, resolving human capital problems, and ensuring accountability and continuity of management.

In our view, independent oversight from an existing IG remains the most effective way to help CSB address its continuing problems, provided that the arrangement is made permanent and funding is provided to the IG for the function.

We are making recommendations to the Chairman of CSB to address continuing problems with governance and management. We are also proposing matters for congressional consideration to address continuing problems with oversight. Regarding the six recommendations, CSB generally concurred with four and disagreed with two. CSB also disagreed with both matters for congressional consideration. CSB did not generally concur with our recommendation to develop a plan to address the investigative gap and request the necessary resources from Congress to meet its statutory mandate but stated that it would work with Congress to clarify the issue of its statutory mandate and, if appropriate, seek an amendment to C SB's authorizing statute.

We believe that CSB's willingness to work with Congress to clarify the issue of its statutory mandate, and if appropriate, seek an amendment to CSB's authorizing statute is a step in the right direction. However, CSB does not agree that it must currently investigate all chemical accidents that meet statutory requirements triggering CSB's responsibility to investigate. In this regard, CSB said it has "not construed the agency's authorizing statute as requiring investigation of every chemical accident involving a fatality, serious injury, or substantial property damage, or the potential for such consequences." We continue to believe the current law is clear; investigations are required for all accidental releases that result, or have the potential to result, in a fatality, serious injury, or substantial property damage. CSB is currently investigating far fewer accidents than is required by law and a plan to address the investigative gap is still necessary.

CSB also disagreed with our recommendation to publish a regulation to require facilities to report information on chemical accidents. We are encouraged that CSB plans to publish in the Federal Register a Request for Information (RFI) concerning a reporting regulation to obtain the views and opinions of CSB's stakeholders. We recognize that this step could provide valuable information regarding the preparation of a reporting regulation. However, the request for information does not in itself provide assurance that CSB will follow through and issue a regulation as required by CSB's authorizing statute. In this regard, CSB said that "a reporting regulation is not needed for the narrow purpose of notifying the CSB of major accidents warranting the deployment of investigators, which appears to be the sole purpose of CSB's authority to issue a reporting rule." We disagree with CSB's view that a reporting regulation is not needed. CSB is legally required to promulgate a regulation. Furthermore, such a regulation would allow CSB to obtain more accurate, complete information to meet its statutory mandate.

In addition, CSB disagreed with our matter for congressional consideration to consider amending CSB's authorizing statute or the Inspector General (IG) Act of 1978 to permanently give EPA's Inspector General the authority to serve as the oversight body for the agency. CSB questioned the independence of the EPA IG, since CSB issues recommendations to EPA. We understand CSB's concerns; however, the IG Act requires inspectors general to be independent from the agencies they audit and investigate, and using the EPA IG does not pose a risk to CSB's independent evaluation of chemical accidents. Finally, CSB disagreed with our matter for congressional consideration to provide the EPA IG with appropriations and staff allocations specifically for the audit of CSB via a direct line in the EPA appropriation. CSB said GAO did not adequately consider different oversight options for CSB and that oversight should be tailored to the size of the agency. We believe that all significant federal programs and entities should be subject to oversight by IGs who can provide sound independent audits of all significant federal operations and activities. The EPA IG has expertise involving the chemical management issues that the Board is charged with investigating, has gained knowledge of CSB's operations and activities in providing the Board with oversight over the past several years, and, like other IGs, has the requisite independence provided by the IG Act of 1978 necessary for reviewing and making recommendations to address long-standing problems in the Board's management performance. Given the management problems that our audit revealed, the need for independent IG oversight at CSB is especially pressing.

August 22, 2008

Congressional Committees

Subject: *Chemical Safety Board: Improvements in Management and Oversight Are Needed*

The principal role of the Chemical Safety and Hazard Investigation Board (CSB) is to investigate accidental releases of regulated or extremely hazardous substances to determine the conditions and circumstances that led to the accident and to identify the cause or causes so that similar accidents might be prevented.[1] Accidental releases of these toxic and hazardous chemicals occur frequently and often have serious consequences. CSB reported to Congress that the agency received notification of approximately 900 chemical accidents in calendar year 2007, and that 31 of these accidents were serious or even fatal events that warranted the commitment of CSB investigators.

CSB began operating in 1998 as an independent agency created under the Clean Air Act Amendments of 1990. The act directs CSB to (1) investigate and report on the cause or probable cause of any accidental chemical releases from stationary sources resulting in a fatality, serious injury, or substantial property damages; (2) make recommendations to reduce the likelihood or consequences of accidental chemical releases and propose corrective measures; and (3) establish regulations for reporting accidental releases. The agency publishes investigative reports and issues safety studies and videos to help prevent future accidents. Congress modeled CSB after the National Transportation Safety Board (NTSB),

---

[1] S. Rpt. No. 101-228, 1990 U.S.C.C.A.N. 3385, 3615 (1989).

which has a similar public safety mission.[2] Like NTSB, CSB has no enforcement authority and a limited regulatory role. As outlined in the authorizing statute, CSB is to be managed by a five-member board. Currently the board has one vacancy. CSB received an appropriation of $9.4 million for fiscal year 2008 and had 39 staff as of January 30, 2008.

In 2000, Congress asked GAO to review CSB's effectiveness in carrying out its mission. In our report, Chemical Safety Board: Improved Policies and Additional Oversight Are Needed (GAO/RCED-00-192),[3] we cited problems with CSB's governance, management, policies, and procedures. Among other things, we recommended that CSB obtain the services of an existing office of inspector general (IG). Since fiscal year 2001, three IGs—from the Federal Emergency Management Agency (FEMA), the Department of Homeland Security (DHS), and the Environmental Protection Agency (EPA)—have provided oversight to CSB. EPA's IG currently provides oversight. Together, over time, these IGs have made 32 recommendations to address problems in management accountability and control, human capital management, compliance with its statutory requirements, and other issues.

In response to a mandate in the Joint Explanatory Statement that accompanied the fiscal year 2008 Consolidated Appropriations Act,[4] we examined (1) how CSB has responded to GAO and IG recommendations regarding CSB's investigative gap, data quality problems, human capital problems, and accountability and management problems for meeting its mission requirements and (2) the merits of the current oversight approach using an existing office of inspector general and other alternative approaches to oversight. On April 17, 2008, we briefed staff from the House and Senate Appropriation Subcommittees on Interior, Environment, and Related Agencies and on May 20, 2008, we briefed the Chairman of the House subcommittee. This letter summarizes the main points from our presentation. See enclosure II for a copy of the briefing slides from that presentation.

---

[2] NTSB is required by statute to investigate every civil aviation accident in the United States and certain railroad, pipeline, and marine accidents and issue safety recommendations aimed at preventing future accidents.
[3] GAO, *Chemical Safety Board: Improved Policies and Additional Oversight Are Needed*, GAO/RCED-00-192 (Washington, D.C.: July 11, 2000).
[4] Joint Explanatory Statement to Accompany the Consolidated Appropriations Amendment, Division F, at 60.

To perform our review, we reviewed relevant documentation and data and interviewed CSB and other agency officials. We conducted this performance audit from October 2007 to May 2008 in accordance with generally accepted government auditing standards. Those standards require that we plan and perform the audit to obtain sufficient, appropriate evidence to provide a reasonable basis for our findings and conclusions based on our audit objectives. We believe that the evidence obtained provides a reasonable basis for our findings and conclusions based on our audit objectives. We determined that the agency's accident-screening database is sufficiently reliable for the purpose of making broad estimates of the total number of accidents and accidents with fatalities. Among the data's limitations is the lack of quality controls to ensure that data are accurate and complete, especially with respect to fatalities. For additional information on our scope and methodology, see enclosure I.

Chapter 1

SUMMARY OF FINDINGS

CSB has implemented some GAO and IG recommendations related to improving its operating policies and procedures since we last reported in July 2000. However, we found that CSB has not fully addressed several critical recommendations, and problems in governance, management, and oversight persist. Specifically, CSB has not fully responded to key recommendations related to investigating more accidents that meet statutory requirements triggering CSB's responsibility to investigate, improving the quality of its accident data, resolving human capital problems, and ensuring accountability and continuity of management.

In our view, independent oversight from an existing IG remains the most effective way to help CSB address its continuing problems, provided that the arrangement is made permanent and funding is provided to the IG for the function.

We are making recommendations to the Chairman of CSB to address continuing problems with governance and management. We are also proposing matters for congressional consideration to address continuing problems with oversight. Regarding the six recommendations, CSB generally concurred with four and disagreed with two. CSB also disagreed with both matters for congressional consideration. CSB did not generally concur with our recommendation to develop a plan to address the investigative gap and request the necessary resources from Congress to meet its statutory mandate but stated that it would work with Congress to clarify the issue of its statutory mandate and, if appropriate, seek an amendment to CSB's authorizing statute. We believe that CSB's willingness to work with Congress to clarify the issue of its statutory mandate, and if appropriate, seek an amendment to CSB's authorizing statute is a step in the right direction. However, CSB does not agree that it must currently investigate all chemical accidents that meet statutory requirements triggering CSB's responsibility to investigate. In this regard, CSB said it has "not construed the agency's authorizing statute as requiring investigation of every chemical accident involving a fatality, serious injury, or substantial property damage, or the potential for such consequences." We continue to believe the current law is clear; investigations are required for all accidental releases that result, or have the potential to result, in a fatality, serious injury, or substantial property damage. CSB is currently investigating far fewer accidents than is required by law and a plan to address the investigative gap is still necessary.

CSB also disagreed with our recommendation to publish a regulation to require facilities to report information on chemical accidents. We are encouraged that CSB plans to publish in the Federal Register a Request for Information (RFI) concerning a reporting regulation to obtain the views and opinions of CSB's stakeholders. We recognize that this step could provide valuable information regarding the preparation of a reporting regulation. However, the request for information does not in itself provide assurance that CSB will follow through and issue a regulation as required by CSB's authorizing statute. In this regard, CSB said that "a reporting regulation is not needed for the narrow purpose of notifying the CSB of major accidents warranting the deployment of investigators, which appears to be the sole purpose of CSB's authority to issue a reporting rule." We disagree with CSB's view that a reporting regulation is not needed. CSB is legally required to promulgate a regulation. Furthermore, such a regulation would allow CSB to obtain more accurate, complete information to meet its statutory mandate.

In addition, CSB disagreed with our matter for congressional consideration to consider amending CSB's authorizing statute or the Inspector General (IG) Act of 1978 to permanently give EPA's Inspector General the authority to serve as the oversight body for the agency. CSB questioned the independence of the EPA IG, since CSB issues recommendations to EPA. We understand CSB's concerns; however, the IG Act requires inspectors general to be independent from the agencies they audit and investigate, and using the EPA IG does not pose a risk to CSB's independent evaluation of chemical accidents.[5] Finally, CSB disagreed with our matter for congressional consideration to provide the EPA IG with appropriations and staff allocations specifically for the audit of CSB via a direct line in the EPA appropriation. CSB said GAO did not adequately consider different oversight options for CSB and that oversight should be tailored to the size of the agency. We believe that all significant federal programs and entities should be subject to oversight by IGs who can provide sound independent audits of all significant federal operations and activities. The EPA IG has expertise involving the chemical management issues that the Board is charged with investigating, has gained knowledge of CSB's operations and activities in providing the Board with oversight over the past several years, and, like other IGs, has the requisite independence provided by the IG Act of 1978 necessary for reviewing and making recommendations to address long-standing problems in the Board's management performance. Given the management problems that our audit revealed, the need for independent IG oversight at CSB is especially pressing.

---

[5] Pub. L. No. 95-452, 92 Stat. 1101 (codified as amended at 5 U.S.C. App. 3).

Chapter 2

CSB HAS NOT FULLY ADDRESSED KEY RECOMMENDATIONS, AND PROBLEMS PERSIST

CSB has not fully responded to recommendations related to its investigative gap, data quality, human capital, and management problems, and we found these problems continue.

THE INVESTIGATIVE GAP PERSISTS

CSB has not fully responded to recommendations to address its investigative gap—the difference between the number of accidents it investigates and the accidents that meet statutory criteria triggering C SB's responsibility to investigate—and this gap persists. Using fiscal year 2002 data, the DHS IG reported in fiscal year 2004 that CSB deployed to 4 of 294 accidents that met statutory criteria for investigation. Moreover, while acknowledging that CSB lacked the resources to investigate all 294 accidents, the IG reported that CSB did not have a plan for reporting to Congress on the number and type of accidents it was not able to investigate, nor did it have a plan for narrowing the investigative gap. Consequently, the IG recommended that CSB develop a plan to describe and address the investigative gap and include the information in future budget submissions to Congress and the Office of Management and Budget (OMB). In response, CSB prepared a onetime report to Congress in 2006. CSB officials told us they did not repeat this report because congressional staff did not request subsequent annual reports with this level of detail. Rather, it included less detailed information in subsequent budget justifications to Congress.

In fiscal year 2007, we found that CSB received notifications of 920 chemical accidents; approximately 35 of these accidents included at least one fatality, and CSB investigated 1 of these. By not investigating all accidental releases that have a fatality, serious injury, substantial property damage, or the potential for a fatality, serious injury, or substantial property damage, CSB continues to fall short of its statutory mandate. CSB officials said the agency lacks the resources to investigate more than a small percentage of the accidents that meet statutory criteria triggering the board's responsibility to investigate. Moreover, CSB has not developed a long-term plan for reporting to Congress on the scope and magnitude of its investigative gap or a detailed strategy to address it. As a result, Congress does not have accurate or comprehensive information about CSB's investigative gap or the resources it would need to close it.

When we compared CSB and NTSB data from 2006, we found that while NTSB's budget is approximately 8 times CSB's budget, NTSB investigates 250 times as many accidents. Unlike CSB, NTSB conducts limited, office-based investigations that rely on the work of other entities. NTSB uses its statutory authority to solicit other entities' work when resources, or other considerations, prevent it from deploying investigators to the accident site, a fact that may help it better leverage its resources. For example, NTSB uses the work of local officials, rescue response units, Federal Aviation Administration (FAA) personnel, and other persons and organizations that might have knowledge of the accident. While CSB has similar statutory authority to use information gathered by others, the agency terminated its limited, office-based review program that relied on other entities work in 1999. Although the limited review program was less resource intensive than full investigations, CSB officials said that they terminated the limited reviews because relying on the work of other agencies conflicted with CSB's independence. In 2006, we reported that NTSB's use of others' work may present some challenges, but appears to be working well.[6] Moreover, CSB has memorandums of understanding with both Occupational Safety and Health Administration (OSHA) and EPA that state that CSB may use information gathered by OSHA and EPA to aid in its investigation of accidents.

DATA QUALITY PROBLEMS CONTINUE

CSB has not fully responded to IG recommendations to publish a data-reporting regulation and improve the quality of its accident data. As a result, data quality problems continue. In 2004, the DHS IG recommended that CSB fulfill its statutory requirement to publish a regulation for receiving information from facilities on their chemical accidents, and that CSB develop a long-term strategy to improve the quality of its data. Since that time, CSB has not issued the regulation, and officials said they have no plans to do so; instead CSB relies primarily on the media, such as online newspapers and television, to learn about chemical accidents. In addition, the DHS IG reported that CSB did not have adequate controls over the quality of data in the accident-screening database it uses to report to Congress and the public on the number of chemical accidents the agency screens and selects for investigation. The IG reported that CSB needed to monitor its data for completeness, accuracy, timeliness, and usefulness.

We found that CSB lacks a long-term strategy to improve quality controls, and the data remain somewhat inaccurate and incomplete. For example, when we analyzed a subset of accidents in the database involving fatalities and injuries, we found at least five accidents (about 6 percent of the cases reviewed) where fatalities were not correctly recorded in the database. We also found seven accidents (about 4 percent of the cases reviewed) where data on injuries were missing as a result of incomplete data entry. Moreover, CSB does not have procedures to ensure that data has been entered accurately. The lack of data-reporting regulations and these data quality problems limit C SB's

---

[6] GAO, *National Transportation Safety Board: Progress Made, Management Practices, Investigation Priorities, and Training Center Use Should Be Improved*, GAO-07-118 (Washington, D.C.: Nov., 22, 2006).

ability to target its resources, identify trends and patterns in chemical accidents, and prevent future similar accidents.

HUMAN CAPITAL PROBLEMS PERSIST

CSB has not fully responded to recommendations to resolve its human capital problems. In 2002, the FEMA IG found that CSB had a shortfall of investigators and had not made hiring them a priority. In addition, it found that CSB lacked a central human capital manager, comprehensive strategic human capital plan, and performance measures and criteria. The FEMA IG recommended that CSB make hiring investigators a top priority and made several recommendations to strengthen its human capital planning and management.

In response, CSB consolidated human capital responsibilities under a full-time human resources manager, developed several agencywide goals to improve human capital, and hired more investigators; however, we found that CSB's human capital strategy was not comprehensive, lacked a detailed action plan for closing the investigator shortfall, did not include input from staff investigators, and lacked performance measures—actions included in the Strategic Management of Human Capital portion of the President's Management Agenda.

CSB officials told us they have difficulties attracting and retaining investigators. We found that more employees left CSB in fiscal years 2006 and 2007 than were hired. In fiscal years 2006 and 2007, three of five investigators who left were senior investigators with 5 to 7 years of experience. Yet CSB hired mostly interns during the same 2 fiscal years. CSB hired these interns through the Federal Career Intern program, which is designed to attract and retain employees for federal service. However, some officials we interviewed, including a board member, investigation managers, and investigators, told us intern investigators are encouraged to leave CSB to gain experience in private industry or to pursue graduate degrees. In addition, CSB officials said they offered retention bonuses to high-performing mid- and senior-level investigators before they left the agency. However, the investigators declined the bonuses because these individuals said they received significantly higher compensation from the private sector. In addition, CSB officials said they did not offer retention bonuses to resigning intern investigators because they did not think it would make a difference since these individuals would be earning more in their new jobs. We found that the agency has not paid a retention bonus to any employee since September 2002. Moreover, we found that in fiscal year 2006, CSB reprogrammed compensation funds of $627,891 to other priorities, including producing safety videos and redesigning its Web site, and that in fiscal year 2007, CSB reprogrammed compensation funds of $407,383 to similar purchases.

ACCOUNTABILITY AND MANAGEMENT PROBLEMS CONTINUE

CSB has not fully responded to recommendations to delegate the authority to effectively manage the day-to-day administrative functions to a permanent chief operating officer (COO). In March 2002, the FEMA IG cited fractured management, a weakened chain of command, and board member intervention in routine administration and recommended that the board delegate day-to-day administrative functions to a permanent COO to ensure continuity of management and accountability. In response to the FEMA IG's recommendation, CSB hired a COO in 2002 to effectively manage the day-to-day operations of CSB, but the individual left in 2004. The board subsequently eliminated the position and transferred the COO's responsibilities to individual program managers and the board.

We found that CSB lacks a permanent senior executive to establish performance goals, hold program mangers accountable for meeting those goals, and demonstrate improvement in the agency's ability to meet its statutory mandate over time. Without a COO, the agency may be unable to ensure continuity of performance and accountability when board members and chairs leave the agency.

CSB board members said that a similar executive director position might reduce the administrative responsibilities of the board; however, in comments to GAO, CSB did not support filling a COO or similar position at this time because a COO is not likely to provide any additional management skills not already represented at the agency. The investigation managers and investigators we interviewed generally expressed support for reinstating the COO position to improve the continuity of administrative management.

Chapter 3

INSPECTOR GENERAL OVERSIGHT IS STILL WARRANTED

On the basis of our review of CSB's history and current operations; we believe that the independent institutional audit presence of an IG remains the best option for ensuring that CSB is accountable to Congress for meeting its statutory requirements. We reconsidered the three options for oversight we suggested in 2000, which include (1) establishing an in-house audit and investigations unit, (2) contracting out for evaluations of its operations and programs, and (3) obtaining the services of an existing office of inspector general. We determined that the first two options are not appropriate for the board for several reasons. The first option—an in-house audit unit—is not practical because CSB's history of management problems warrants a level of independent oversight that may be difficult to achieve by an internal audit function. In addition, the limited staffing that would reasonably be allocated to this function at an agency of this size would lack the varied expertise needed to address these problems. The second option—contracting out for evaluations—is not appropriate because of the limitations of contracting in terms of both audit independence and the potentially limited duration of the contracting relationship. CSB officials told us they prefer the second option because they believe CSB's small size does not justify independent institutional IG oversight. In addition, CSB officials said that CSB is classified as one of 54 federal entities defined in the IG Act of 1978 for which the act did not provide an IG, but rather required annual reporting of their audit and investigative activities to Congress and the Office of Management and Budget. However, in our view, the CSB's long-standing, serious, and intractable management problems make it unlikely that the reporting requirements for federal entities will ensure that the CSB has an appropriate level of oversight to address its management problems.

Given these factors, in our view IG oversight remains the most appropriate oversight option for CSB. Nonetheless, we recognize that there are some shortcomings with the current EPA IG's oversight relationship. First, the arrangement is not permanent, a fact that may undermine the continuity of oversight. Second, EPA IG officials told us they have no plans to conduct future program evaluations of CSB because they are allocating their limited evaluation resources to other priority issues within EPA. However, we do not believe, as CSB asserts, that the EPA IG's assignment and work call into question CSB's intended independence from EPA. According to CSB, CSB independently evaluates and reports to Congress on EPA programs in chemical accident prevention, and CSB's independence from EPA was deliberate and carefully considered. By statute, inspectors general are independent from the agencies they audit and investigate so the EPA IG must maintain his or her independence from EPA officials and program employees. With such independence, the IG poses no risk to CSB's independent evaluations of chemical accidents.

Chapter 4

CONCLUSIONS

After 10 years of operation, CSB continues to operate in noncompliance with its statutory mandates. CSB stresses that it recognizes the importance of its investigations to identify root causes of accidental releases and recommend regulatory action to prevent such accidental releases, but it is not investigating all chemical releases that have a fatality, serious injury, substantial property damage, or the potential for a fatality, serious injury, or substantial property damage.

Given the resource constraints on the board that limit its ability to investigate all chemical accidents resulting in f, serious injuries, or substantial property damage, it is particularly important that CSB better leverage its existing resources by using other entities' work, have the best available data on which to make decisions on those accidents that are most important to investigate, and use all available human capital tools to retain staff. Even though CSB has a statutory requirement to issue a regulation requiring facilities to report their chemical releases, the board has resisted requiring such reporting, preferring to rely on alternative information sources, such as major news organizations. Requiring facilities to report certain information on accidental releases would provide CSB with better data than it currently receives from media sources.

The difficulties that CSB has experienced are largely the result of inadequate management accountability for addressing long-standing problems and for clearly identifying and attempting to meet CSB's staff requirements to perform investigations of chemical accidents. While we recognize that CSB may not have sufficient resources to investigate every accident within its purview, as NTSB reports it does, we believe CSB is missing opportunities to investigate more accidents and possibly prevent fatalities, serious injuries, and substantial property damage in the future. For example, other federal agencies, such as EPA and OSHA, collect accident information that, to the extent that the information meets CSB's data quality standards, could provide additional resources to help the board meet its mission.

Chapter 5

RECOMMENDATIONS FOR EXECUTIVE ACTION

We recommend that the chairman of the Chemical Safety Board

- develop a plan to address the investigative gap and request the necessary resources from Congress to meet CSB's statutory mandate or seek an amendment to its statutory mandate;
- consider using the work of other entities, such as government agencies, companies, and contractors (subject to an assessment of the quality of their work), to a greater extent to maximize the board's limited resources;
- improve the quality of its accident-screening database by better controlling data entry and periodically sampling accident data to evaluate their consistency and completeness;
- publish a regulation requiring facilities to report all chemical accidents, as required by law, to better inform the agency of important details about accidents that it may not receive from current sources;
- consider reinstating the position of chief operating officer, with delegations of responsibility for establishing performance goals, holding program mangers accountable for meeting those goals, and demonstrating improvement in the agency's ability to meet it statutory mandates over time; and

- use the Strategic Management of Human Capital portion of the President's Management Agenda to provide criteria for developing a comprehensive human capital plan, with input from investigators that includes specific objectives and performance measures to improve accountability for results and to assist the agency in its goal of improving its human capital and infrastructure.

Chapter 6

MATTERS FOR CONGRESSIONAL CONSIDERATION

Congress may wish to consider amending CSB's authorizing statute or the Inspector General Act of 1978 to permanently give EPA's Inspector General the authority to serve as the oversight body for the agency.

As Congress prepares the appropriation of the EPA Inspector General, it may wish to consider providing the Inspector General with appropriations and staff allocations specifically for the audit function of CSB via a direct line in the EPA appropriation.

Chapter 7

AGENCY COMMENTS AND OUR EVALUATION

We provided a draft of our report to CSB for its review and comment. We received written comments from CSB's Chairman and Chief Executive Officer (CEO). These comments and our detailed response to them are presented in enclosure III. CSB also provided technical comments, which we have incorporated into the report as appropriate.

Regarding the six specific recommendations we made in the report, CSB generally concurred with four and disagreed with two. CSB also disagreed with both matters for congressional consideration we identified in the report. CSB generally concurred that it should (1) consider using the work of other entities to maximize the board's limited resources, (2) improve the quality of its accident-screening database, (3) consider reinstating the position of chief operating officer, (4) use the Strategic Management of Human Capital portion of the President's Management Agenda as a guide for developing a comprehensive human capital plan.

CSB did not generally concur with our recommendation to develop a plan to address the investigative gap and request the necessary resources from Congress to meet its statutory mandate. The agency reports that it will seek additional investigation resources and "will draft a plan for obtaining information on additional chemical accidents occurring in the United States, and clearly set forth a risk-based approach to accident selection and investigation." However, it does not commit to meet CSB's statutory mandate for investigating chemical releases, citing its view that "CSB has not construed the agency's authorizing statute as requiring investigation of every chemical accident involving a fatality, serious injury, or substantial property damage, or the potential for such consequences." CSB has not explained the basis for its interpretation. The 1990 Clean Air Act Amendments establishing the CSB states "[t]he Board shall investigate (or cause to be investigated)... any accidental release resulting in a fatality, serious injury or substantial property damage." Further, the act states that "[i]n no event shall the Board forgo an investigation where an accidental release causes a fatality or serious injury among the general public, or had [sic] the potential to cause substantial property damage or a number of deaths or injuries among the general public." As noted in our briefing, this language clearly identifies which accidental releases CSB is required to investigate; that is, investigations are required for all accidental releases that result, or have the potential to result, in a fatality, serious injury, or substantial property damage. Although CSB did not agree with this interpretation, the agency stated that it would work with Congress to clarify the issue of its statutory mandate and, if appropriate, seek an amendment to CSB's authorizing statute. We believe that CSB's willingness to work with Congress to clarify its statutory mandate is a step in the right direction. However, we continue to believe the current law is clear; CSB should meet its current mandate or seek an amendment to its authorizing statute.

CSB disagreed with our matter for congressional consideration to consider amending CSB's authorizing statute or the IG Act of 1978 to permanently give EPA's Inspector General the authority to serve as the oversight body for the agency. CSB said that while the EPA IG is one option for oversight, other offices of inspector general are also available, some of which may be more appropriate for the role. CSB also questioned the independence of the EPA IG, since CSB issues recommendations to EPA program offices. We assessed other options for oversight that we had considered in our 2000 report, as well as options presented to us by CSB. We understand CSB's concerns; however, the IG Act requires inspectors general to be independent from the agencies they audit and investigate. The EPA IG has expertise involving the chemical management issues that the Board is charged with investigating, has gained knowledge of CSB's operations and activities in providing the Board with oversight over the past several years, and, like other IGs, has the requisite independence provided by the IG Act of 1978 necessary for reviewing and making recommendations to address long-standing problems in the Board's management performance. As a result, using the EPA IG does not pose a risk to CSB's independent evaluation of chemical accidents.

CSB also disagreed with our matter for congressional consideration to provide the EPA IG with appropriations and staff allocations specifically for the audit of CSB via a direct line in the EPA appropriation. CSB said GAO did not adequately consider different oversight options for CSB and that oversight should be tailored to the size of the agency. CSB also noted that it currently obtains its financial and information security audits for about $60,000 a year. We believe that all significant federal programs and entities should be subject to oversight by IGs who can provide sound independent audits of all significant federal operations and activities. Given the management problems that our audit revealed, the need for independent IG oversight at CSB is especially pressing. Further, financial and information security audits are not a substitute for the oversight of program management provided by an independent IG.

We are sending copies of this report to the Chairman and CEO of the Chemical Safety and Hazard Investigation Board, appropriate congressional committees, and other interested parties. We will also make copies available to others upon request. In addition, the report will be available at no charge on the GAO Web site at http://www.gao.gov.

If you or your staff have any questions about this report, please contact me at 202-512-3841 or stephensonj@gao.gov. Contact points for our Offices of Congressional Relations and Public Affairs may be found on the last page of this report. Major contributors to this report were Ed Kratzer, Assistant Director; Vanessa Dillard; Brian M. Friedman; Angela Miles; Alison O'Neill; Michael Sagalow; Rebecca Shea; John C. Smith; and Jeanette Soares.

John B. Stephenson
Director, Natural Resources and Environment

Enclosures

> *Congressional Addressees*
> The Honorable Dianne Feinstein
> Chairman
> The Honorable Wayne Allard
> Ranking Member
> Subcommittee on Interior, Environment, and Related Agencies
> Committee on Appropriations
> United States Senate
> The Honorable Norman D. Dicks
> Chairman

The Honorable Todd Tiahrt
Ranking Member
Subcommittee on Interior, Environment, and Related Agencies
Committee on Appropriations
House of Representatives

ENCLOSURE I. SCOPE AND METHODOLOGY

To perform our review, we analyzed authorizing statutes, regulations, legislative history, and GAO and office of inspector general (IG) reports, and other literature. We also reviewed and analyzed the Chemical Safety and Hazard Investigation Board's (CSB) strategic plan, human capital report, policies and procedures, and other program documents, and compared them to similar documents from the National Transportation Safety Board (NTSB). In addition, we reviewed a subset of CSB's accident screening database that included two variables CSB uses to rank the seriousness of an accident—fatalities and injuries and the narratives explaining these accidents. We also consulted GAO's guidance on management best practices, human capital, data reliability, and oversight. In addition, we interviewed officials from CSB, officials from past and current IGs. We also consulted NTSB officials and GAO experts on management, data reliability, human capital, and oversight issues.

We did not evaluate the quality of CSB's investigative products issued to date, or the quality and effectiveness of its reports, recommendations, and promotion of preventive actions, because these evaluations were outside the scope of our mandate and are not relevant to the findings and conclusions of this engagement. We also did not conduct a detailed evaluation of the oversight arrangements for the other 53 federal entities for comparison with CSB because the continuing management problems found in our audit highlight the need for IG oversight.

We conducted this performance audit from October 2007 to May 2008 in accordance with generally accepted government auditing standards. Those standards require that we plan and perform the audit to obtain sufficient, appropriate evidence to provide a reasonable basis for our findings and conclusions based on our audit objectives. We believe that the evidence obtained provides a reasonable basis for our findings and conclusions based on our audit objectives. We determined that the agency's accident screening database is sufficiently reliable for the purpose of making broad estimates of the total number of accidents and accidents with fatalities. Among the data's limitations is the lack of quality controls to ensure that data are accurate and complete, especially with respect to fatalities.

ENCLOSURE II. SLIDES FROM APRIL 17, 2008, BRIEFING TO CONGRESSIONAL STAFF

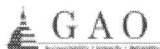

Chemical Safety Board: Improvements in Management and Oversight Are Needed

Briefing to the Subcommittees on Interior, Environment, and Related Agencies,
Committee on Appropriations,
U.S. Senate
U.S. House of Representatives

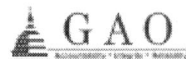

Background

- The Chemical Safety and Hazard Investigation Board (CSB) is an independent agency that was created under the Clean Air Act Amendments of 1990 and began operating in 1998. The act directed CSB to
  - investigate and report on the cause or probable cause of any accidental chemical releases resulting in a fatality, a serious injury, or substantial property damage;
  - make recommendations to reduce the likelihood or consequences of accidental chemical releases and propose corrective measures; and
  - establish regulations for reporting accidental releases.

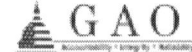

Background

- Congress modeled CSB after the National Transportation Safety Board (NTSB), which has a similar mission.
- Like NTSB, CSB has no enforcement authority and a limited regulatory role.
- As outlined in the statute, CSB is to be managed by a five-member board. Currently the board has one vacancy.
- In fiscal year 2009, CSB requested $10.6 million and 47 staff.
- In fiscal year 2000, CSB requested $12.5 million and 60 staff.
- Prior year appropriations and on-board staff levels include
  - fiscal year 2008, $9.4 million and 39 staff (as of 1/30/2008);
  - fiscal year 2006, $9.2 million and 41 staff (as of 9/30/2006);
  - fiscal year 2004, $8.2 million and 40 staff (as of 9/30/2004); and
  - fiscal year 2000, $8.0 million and 27 staff (as of 6/15/2000).

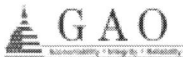

Background

- In 2000, GAO reported problems with CSB's governance, management, policies, and procedures and recommended, among other things, that CSB obtain the services of an existing office of inspector general (IG).
- Since fiscal year 2001, three existing IGs have provided oversight to CSB: Federal Emergency Management Agency (FEMA), the Department of Homeland Security (DHS), and the U.S. Environmental Protection Agency (EPA). EPA's IG currently provides oversight.
- From fiscal year 2002 through 2007, inspectors general have made 32 recommendations to address problems in management accountability and control, human capital management, compliance with its statutory requirements, and other issues.

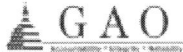

Objectives

- You asked us to examine
    1. how CSB has responded to GAO and IG recommendations regarding CSB's investigative gap, data quality problems, human capital problems, and accountability and management problems for meeting its mission requirements and
    2. the merits of the current oversight approach—using an existing office of inspector general—and other alternative approaches to oversight.

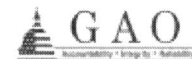

Scope and Methodology

- To answer these questions, we reviewed
  - authorizing statutes, regulations, legislative history and GAO and IG reports, and other literature;
  - CSB's accident screening database for fiscal year 2006 and fiscal year 2007;
  - CSB's strategic plan, human capital report, and other program documentation such as policies and procedures;
  - similar program documents from NTSB for comparison to CSB documents;
  - GAO guidance pertaining to management best practices, human capital, data reliability, and oversight; and
  - The mission and oversight arrangements for 54 federal entities, including CSB, as defined by the Inspector General Act of 1978.
- We did not review or evaluate the quality or effectiveness CSB's products, recommendations or preventive actions as that was outside the scope of our mandate and not relevant to this engagement's findings and conclusions.

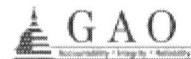

Scope and Methodology

- We also interviewed officials from CSB and past and current IGs and consulted GAO experts on management, data reliability, human capital, and oversight issues.
- We conducted this performance audit from October 2007 to May 2008 in accordance with generally accepted government auditing standards. Those standards require that we plan and perform the audit to obtain sufficient, appropriate evidence to provide a reasonable basis for our findings and conclusions based on our audit objectives. We believe that the evidence obtained provides a reasonable basis for our findings and conclusions based on our audit objectives. We determined that the agency's accident-screening database is sufficiently reliable for the purpose of making broad estimates of the total number of accidents and accidents with fatalities. Among the data's limitations is the lack of quality controls to ensure that data are accurate and complete, especially with respect to fatalities.

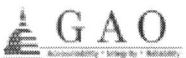

Results in Brief

- CSB has implemented some GAO and IG recommendations related to improving its operating policies and procedures since we last reported in July 2000. However, CSB has not fully addressed several critical recommendations, and problems in governance, management, and oversight persist. Specifically, CSB has not fully responded to key recommendations related to (1) investigating more accidents that meet statutory requirements triggering the CSB's responsibility to investigate, (2) improving the quality of its accident data, (3) resolving human capital problems, and (4) ensuring accountability and continuity of management.
- In our view, independent oversight from an existing IG remains the most effective way to help CSB address its continuing problems, provided that the arrangement is made permanent and funding is provided to the IG for the function. CSB officials disagreed based on the agency's small size and its existing annual reporting requirements to Congress and the Office of Management and Budget.
- Therefore
  - We are making recommendations to the Chair of CSB to address continuing problems with governance and management.
  - We are proposing matters for congressional consideration to address continuing problems with oversight.

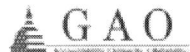

The investigative gap persists

- CSB has not fully responded to recommendations to address its investigative gap—the difference between the number of accidents it investigates and the accidents that meet statutory criteria triggering CSB's responsibility to investigate.
- <u>Initial problem</u>: Using fiscal year 2002 data, the DHS IG reported in fiscal year 2004 that of the 613 accidents CSB screened, about 294 met statutory criteria, and CSB deployed investigators to 4. Moreover, while acknowledging that CSB lacked the resources to investigate all 294 accidents, the IG reported that CSB did not have a plan for reporting to Congress on the number and type of accidents it was not able to investigate or a plan for narrowing the investigative gap.

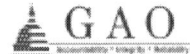

The investigative gap persists

- <u>IG's recommendation</u>: The DHS IG recommended that CSB develop a plan to describe and address the investigative gap and include the information in future budget submissions to Congress and OMB.
- <u>How CSB responded</u>: Two years after the IG made the recommendation, CSB prepared a onetime report to Congress in 2006. The report described 14 accidents occurring in 1 year that it said it would have investigated if it had had the resources. However, the report did not describe a plan to address the investigative gap identified by DHS IG.
    - CSB has not repeated this report; rather, it included less detailed information in subsequent budget justifications to Congress.
    - CSB officials told us that congressional staff did not request subsequent annual reports with this level of detail.
    - CSB officials also said the agency lacks the resources to investigate more than a small percentage of the accidents that meet statutory criteria triggering the board's responsibility to investigate.

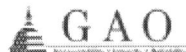

The investigative gap persists

- <u>Problem remaining</u>: CSB continues to underestimate the number of accidents it would need to investigate to meet statutory requirements. In addition, it has not significantly narrowed its investigative gap—investigating about 6 accidents each year from fiscal years 2004 through 2007. Moreover, CSB has not developed a long-term plan for reporting to Congress on the scope and magnitude of its investigative gap or a detailed strategy to address it. Therefore
    - CSB continues to fall short of its statutory mandate, and accidents that involve fatalities, serious injuries, and substantial property damage go uninvestigated.
    - Congress does not have accurate or comprehensive information about CSB's investigative gap or the resources it would need to close it.

Enclosure II: Slides from April 17, 2008, Briefing to Congressional Staff 35

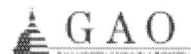

The investigative gap persists

- In fiscal year 2007, CSB investigated less than 1 percent (5 of 920) of accidents of which it was notified.
- Examples of accidents in fiscal years 2006 and 2007 that CSB did not investigate include
  - An oil well explosion that killed 3 teens.
  - A methanol flash fire at a school that injured 8 students and their teacher. Three students and the teacher were hospitalized for burns on their upper torsos, faces, and hands.
  - A natural gas well explosion that killed 1 worker and forced hundreds of residents out of their homes for hours.
  - A propane explosion that killed 3 workers and injured 47.
  - A waste-processing plant that released noxious chemicals and may have sickened more than 200 people.

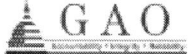

The investigative gap persists

Table 1: Information on Chemical Accidents and Investigations, Fiscal Years 2006 and 2007

	2006	2007
Total accidents CSB recorded in its screening database	822[a]	920[a]
Accidents CSB deployed to	9[b]	8[b]
Accidents CSB investigated	6	5
Accidents with fatalities	38[a]	35[a]
Accidents with fatalities that CSB investigated	5	1

Source: GAO analysis of CSB data.

[a] Because of data quality limitations, the total number of accidents and accidents with fatalities identified and reported in the database may be underestimated.

[b] The number of deployments is greater than the number of accident investigations because CSB deployed to accidents it did not ultimately investigate.

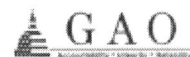

The investigative gap persists

- CSB and NTSB are both required to investigate all accidents meeting certain criteria. NTSB is required to investigate (1) all civil aviation accidents; (2) all pipeline accidents in which there is a fatality, substantial property damage, or significant injury to the environment; (3) all railroad accidents in which there is a fatality or substantial property damage, or that involves a passenger train; and (4) certain major marine casualties. Likewise, CSB is required to investigate all accidental chemical releases into the air from stationary sources that cause a fatality, serious injury, or substantial property damage. NTSB does have discretion in selecting which highway and "other modes of transportation" accidents to investigate. CSB's authorizing statute does not give it any discretion in selecting which accidents to investigate.
- While NTSB's budget is approximately 8 times CSB's budget, NTSB investigates 250 times as many accidents.
- Figure 1 describes the annual budget and the number of investigations CSB and NTSB started in fiscal year 2006.

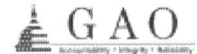

The investigative gap persists

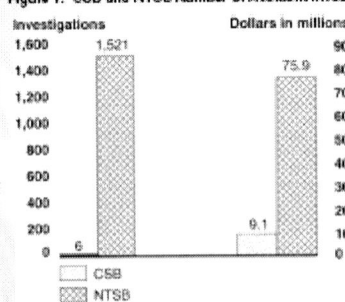

Figure 1. CSB and NTSB Number of Accident Investigations Initiated and Budget, fiscal year 2006

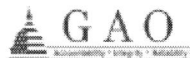

The investigative gap persists

- Both CSB's and NTSB's statutes allow the use of investigations performed by other agencies. Unlike CSB, NTSB uses its authority to solicit investigative work performed by others when resources or other considerations prevent it from deploying to accident sites. In all cases, overall investigative control, including determination of probable cause, rests with NTSB.
- NTSB's size prevents it from being on-site for many aviation investigations; therefore, the agency conducts limited investigations in which NTSB investigators do not go to the scene of the accident to gather information but rather correspond with local officials, rescue response units, Federal Aviation Administration personnel, and other persons and organizations that might have knowledge of the accident. The different types of NTSB aviation investigations are described in attachment 2.
- Similar to NTSB, CSB has the authority to use information gathered by local officials, rescue response units, Occupational Safety & Health Administration (OSHA) and EPA personnel, and other persons and organizations to prepare its reports and thereby expand its knowledge base of chemical accidents while operating with limited resources.

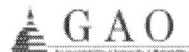

The investigative gap persists

- CSB has memorandums of understanding with OSHA and EPA that indicate in certain instances, CSB may decide not to send an investigation team to the site of a chemical incident but may collect incident information from EPA, OSHA, or other on-site agencies compiled in the course of their own actions.
- Like NTSB, CSB has the ability to issue accident briefs, in addition to more detailed accident reports. See attachment 3 for a description of the types of NTSB accident reports.

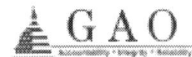

The investigative gap persists

- We reported in 2000 that CSB discontinued its limited, office-based review program that used investigative reports prepared by other organizations that respond to accidents. While the limited review program was less resource intensive than full investigations, board officials told us that they terminated this practice in 1999 because it conflicted with the board's independence by having the board rely on the work of other agencies.
- In contrast, NTSB does conduct limited, office-based investigations that rely on the work of other entities. We reported in 2006 that while NTSB's use of others' work may present some challenges, it appears to be working well. Performing data reliability assessments of important information based on the work of others is a generally accepted means used by federal and private audit organizations. CSB could likewise use existing reports and studies rather than performing comprehensive investigations of its own.

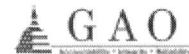

Data quality problems continue

- CSB has not fully responded to IG recommendations to improve the quality of its accident data.
- <u>Initial problem</u>: CSB maintains an accident-screening database to report to Congress and the public on the number of chemical accidents it identifies and selects for investigation. However, the Department of Homeland Security (DHS) IG reported that CSB had inadequate control over the quality of its data and needed to monitor for completeness, accuracy, timeliness, and usefulness.

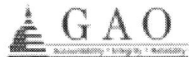

Data quality problems continue

- <u>The IG's recommendation</u>: The DHS IG recommended that CSB fulfill its statutory requirement to publish a regulation for receiving information from facilities on their chemical accidents. The IG also recommended that CSB develop a long-term strategy to address the shortfall in national chemical accident database quality.
- <u>How CSB responded</u>: CSB has not issued the regulation and has no plans to do so. According to CSB officials, the current system of monitoring media reports, searching the Web, and obtaining accident reports from NTSB and other sources is sufficient.

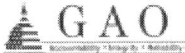

Data quality problems continue

- <u>Problem remaining</u>: According to CSB officials, they have resolved the IG's concerns about data quality; however, we found that CSB still has not published a data-reporting regulation and lacks a long-term strategy to improve quality controls, and the data remain somewhat inaccurate and incomplete. For example, when we analyzed a subset of accidents in the database involving fatalities and injuries, we found at least five accidents (about 6 percent) where fatalities were not correctly recorded in the database. We also found seven accidents (about 4 percent) where data on injuries were missing as a result of incomplete data entry. Moreover, CSB does not have procedures to ensure that data were entered accurately.

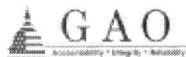

Data quality problems continue

- CSB officials maintain that publishing a regulation to obtain information from facilities on their chemical accidents is not necessary because the information the board already receives is sufficient. Without a regulation, CSB relies primarily on the media, such as online newspapers and television, to learn about chemical accidents. It is likely that information reported by facilities would be a better source than CSB's current practice of relying mostly on the media. Information provided in media sources may contain errors and not include the kind of information CSB needs to make decisions about which accidents to investigate or provide the agency with the kind of information needed for trend analysis and prevention outreach.
- In addition, the lack of quality controls of CSB's accident database has contributed to data problems that could limit CSB's ability to accurately report information on the investigative gap to Congress, target its resources, identify trends and patterns in chemical accidents, and prevent future similar accidents.

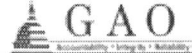

Human capital problems persist

- CSB has not fully responded to recommendations to resolve its human capital problems.
- <u>Initial problem</u>: In 2002, the FEMA IG identified weaknesses in CSB's human capital management, particularly that it had a shortfall of investigators, had not made hiring investigators a top priority, and that it lacked a central human capital manager, a comprehensive strategic human capital plan, and performance measures and criteria.

Enclosure II: Slides from April 17, 2008, Briefing to Congressional Staff

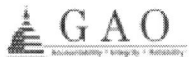

Human capital problems persist

- <u>IG's recommendation</u>: The FEMA IG recommended that CSB make hiring a top priority and made several recommendations to strengthen its human capital planning and management.
- <u>How CSB responded</u>: CSB consolidated human capital responsibilities under a full-time human resources manager, developed several agencywide strategies that included goals to improve human capital, hired more investigators, and established a remote office in Denver for one senior investigation manager. However, CSB officials acknowledged difficulties in attracting senior investigators to live in the District of Columbia and in retaining intern investigators.

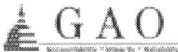

Human capital problems persist

- <u>Problem remaining</u>: CSB's human capital strategy was not comprehensive, lacked a detailed action plan for closing the investigator shortfall, did not include input from staff investigators, and lacked performance measures—actions included in the Strategic Management of Human Capital portion of the President's Management Agenda. Therefore
    - CSB's shortfall in investigators and problems retaining staff continue, limiting the number of accidents CSB could investigate regardless of resources.
    - According to a board member and some investigation managers and investigators we interviewed, intern investigators are encouraged to leave CSB in order to gain private industry experience or to pursue a terminal graduate degree. Encouraging interns to leave federal service for private industry experience does not follow the purpose of the Federal Career Intern program, which is designed to attract and retain employees for federal service.

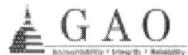

Human capital problems persist

- More employees left CSB in fiscal years 2006 and 2007 than were hired, indicating a possible problem with retention.
- CSB officials acknowledge a problem with hiring and retention; however, the agency has not given a retention bonus to an employee since 2002.

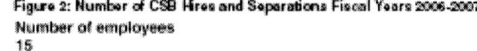

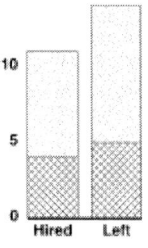

Figure 2: Number of CSB Hires and Separations Fiscal Years 2006-2007

Noninvestigative staff
Investigators

Source: CSB's budget and staffing plan documents.

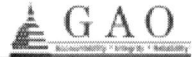

Human capital problems persist

- In fiscal years 2006 and 2007, 3 of 5 investigators who left CSB were senior investigators with 5-7 years of experience. Yet CSB hired mostly interns during the same 2 fiscal years.
- In fiscal years 2006 and 2007, 4 of 11 staff hired were investigators. Three of the 4 investigators CSB hired were interns. CSB officials told us that they can hire interns more easily than senior investigators.

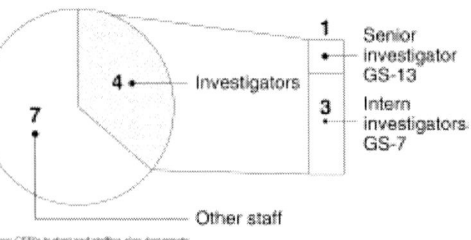

Figure 3: CSB Investigators and Other Staff Hired, Fiscal Years 2006–2007

1 Senior investigator GS-13
3 Intern investigators GS-7
4 Investigators
7 Other staff

Source: CSB's budget and staffing plan documents.

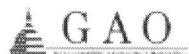

Human capital problems persist

- According to CSB officials, an intern does not replace an experienced senior investigator; after converting to a permanent position from the intern position, it takes 3 to 5 years to become fully qualified.
- However, CSB officials said retaining interns is a challenge and noted that two of four intern investigators hired in fiscal years 2004 and 2005 left CSB and one transferred to another office.
- If CSB had retained intern investigators hired in fiscal years 2004 and 2005, it would have two additional investigators with 3 years of experience in fiscal year 2008.

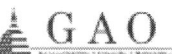

Human capital problems persist

- CSB has not fully used strategies available to federal agencies that are designed to recruit or retain staff, such as
    - Federal Career Intern Program—The purpose of the federal intern program is to convert successful interns to permanent employees. The majority of interns have left CSB.
    - Education and training assistance—Intern investigators interested in pursuing a graduate degree might remain at CSB if the agency offered support for tuition and additional training.
    - Retention bonuses—Federal agencies may pay a retention incentive to a current employee if the agency determines that it is essential to retain the employee. CSB has not given any employee a retention bonus since September 2002.
    - Remote offices—CSB has not expanded the use of remote offices.

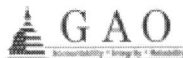

Human capital problems persist

- In fiscal year 2006, CSB reprogrammed compensation funds of $627,891 to other priorities, such as safety videos and redesigning a Web site. In fiscal year 2007, CSB reprogrammed compensation funds of $407,383 to similar purchases.
- Had CSB made resolving human capital problems a top priority, these funds could have been used during the year for recruitment and retention bonuses, education and training assistance, and student loan repayment to hire and retain investigators.

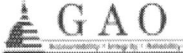

Accountability and management problems continue

- CSB has not delegated the authority to effectively manage the day-to-day administrative functions to a permanent chief operating officer (COO) to ensure continuity of management and accountability.
- <u>Initial problem</u>: Between fiscal years 2000 and 2002, CSB did not have a permanent COO or a fully staffed board with a chair. Uncertainties surrounding the acting COO's role and authority resulted in fractured management, a weakened chain of command, and board member intervention in routine administration.

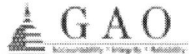

Accountability and management problems continue

- <u>IG's recommendation</u>: The IG recommended that the board delegate to the COO the authority to effectively manage the day-to-day operations of CSB.
- <u>How CSB responded</u>: CSB hired a COO in June 2002, but the individual left after 2 years. The board subsequently eliminated the position and transferred the COO's responsibilities to individual program managers and the board.
  - CSB board members said that a COO or similar executive director position might reduce the administrative responsibilities of the board; however, the CSB Chairman said a COO is unlikely to provide any additional management skills not already represented at the agency. Two investigation managers and two investigators we interviewed generally expressed support for reinstating the COO position to improve the continuity of administrative management.
  - EPA IG officials told us that there was support for the COO position among the CSB employees (former and current) they interviewed during their investigation in fiscal year 2007. These CSB employees indicated that they preferred how things operated when the COO was present.

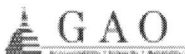

Accountability and management problems continue

- <u>Problem remaining</u>: CSB continues to operate without a permanent COO or a fully staffed board. Therefore
  - CSB lacks a permanent senior executive with responsibility to establish performance goals, hold program managers accountable for meeting those goals, ensure there is a shared vision among board members and managers, and demonstrate improvement in the agency's ability to meet it statutory mission over time.
  - CSB may not be able to ensure continuity of performance and accountability when board members and chairs leave the agency.
  - Regardless of the board's staffing status, GAO has recommended in the past that employing a COO would provide long-term attention and focus on management issues.

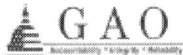

IG oversight is still warranted

- CSB's history suggests that an IG's continued independent institutional audit presence is the best option for ensuring that CSB is more accountable to Congress for meeting its public safety mission and statutory requirements.
  As we reported in 2000, three options for oversight include
  1. establishing an in-house audit and investigations unit,
  2. contracting out for evaluations of its operations and programs, and
  3. obtaining the services of an existing office of inspector general.
- We do not believe options 1 and 2 are appropriate for the board for several reasons.

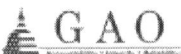

IG oversight is still warranted

- Option 1, an in-house audit unit, does not appear to be practical because CSB's history of management problems warrants a level of independent oversight that may be difficult to achieve by an internal audit function. In addition, the limited staffing that would reasonably be allocated to this function at an agency of this size would lack the varied expertise need to address these problems.
- Option 2, contracting out for evaluations, also does not appear to be appropriate because of the limitations of contracting in terms of both audit independence and the potentially limited duration of the contracting relationship—which would not provide the continuity of oversight needed to address CSB's long-standing management problems.

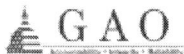

IG oversight is still warranted

- CSB officials told us they prefer option 2 because IG oversight is inappropriate for an agency of CSB's small size. CSB officials told us that CSB is currently classified as 1 of 54 federal entities, as defined by the IG Act of 1978, for which the act did not provide an IG.
  - Under the IG Act, federal entities are required to report annually to Congress and the Office of Management and Budget on whether an IG has been established or what other actions the federal entity took to otherwise ensure that audits of its programs and operations were conducted.
- CSB officials also told us that the IG Act provides a reasonable and responsible level of oversight for federal entities and requested that CSB be treated similarly to these entities. However, in our view, CSB's long-standing, serious, and intractable management problems make it unlikely that this reporting requirement alone will ensure that the CSB has an appropriate level of oversight necessary to address its management problems.

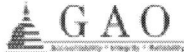

IG oversight is still warranted

- Given CSB's management problems, the fact that other federal entities lack an IG should not determine whether CSB should have an IG. In any event, by statute some other federal entities do have another agency's IG assigned to provide them with oversight. For example, the IG of the Department of Agriculture is assigned to provide oversight to the Delta Regional Authority. (Att. 1 provides the list of 54 federal entities, as defined by the IG Act of 1978, and identifies 4 that have a critical safety mission.)

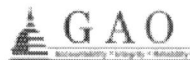

IG oversight is still warranted

- Option 3, obtaining the services of an existing IG office, appears to be the most appropriate oversight arrangement given the serious, intractable management problems at CSB.
- We believe that all significant federal programs and entities should be subject to oversight by IGs who can provide sound independent audits of all significant federal operations and activities. Given the management problems that our audit revealed, the need for independent IG oversight is especially pressing.

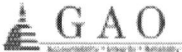

IG oversight is still warranted

- While we believe that IG oversight remains the most appropriate oversight option, we found some shortcomings with the current EPA IG's oversight relationship:
    - The current IG arrangement is not permanent, a fact that may undermine the continuity of oversight; the EPA IG is assigned to serve as CSB's IG in annual appropriation bills.
    - EPA IG officials told us they have no plans to conduct program evaluations of CSB in fiscal year 2008 because they are allocating their limited evaluation resources to other priorities within EPA.
- However, we do not believe, as CSB asserts, that the EPA IG's assignment and work call into question CSB's intended independence from EPA. According to CSB, CSB independently evaluates and reports to Congress on EPA programs in chemical accident prevention and CSB's independence from EPA was deliberate and carefully considered. By statute, inspectors general are independent from the agencies they audit and investigate so the EPA IG must maintain his or her independence from EPA officials and program employees. With such independence, the IG poses no risk to CSB's independent evaluations of chemical accidents.

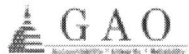

Conclusions

- After 10 years of operation, CSB continues to operate in noncompliance with its statutory mandates.
- CSB stresses that it recognizes the importance of its investigations to identify root causes of accidental releases and recommend regulatory action to prevent such accidental releases but is not investigating all chemical accidents that have a fatality, serious injury, property damage, or the potential for a fatality, serious injury, or property damage.
- While we recognize that CSB may not have sufficient resources to investigate every accident within its purview, as NTSB reports it does, we believe CSB is missing opportunities to investigate more accidents and possibly prevent fatalities, serious injuries, and substantial property damage in the future by not using the work of other entities.

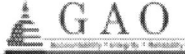

Conclusions

- In addition, given the resource constraints on the board that limit its ability to investigate all chemical accidents resulting in fatalities, serious injuries, or substantial property damage, it is particularly important that CSB have the best available data on which to make decisions on those accidents that are most important to investigate. Even though CSB has a statutory requirement to issue a regulation requiring facilities to report their chemical releases, the board has resisted requiring such reporting, preferring to rely on alternative information sources, such as major news organizations.
- The difficulties that CSB has experienced in meeting its mission are largely the result of inadequate management accountability for addressing long-standing problems and for clearly identifying and attempting to meet CSB's staff requirements to perform investigations of chemical accidents. In this regard, CSB has functioned without a permanent chief operations officer with responsibility for holding CSB's managers accountable for their management activities and has not developed a comprehensive human capital strategy to improve its efforts to investigate chemical accidents in line with the board's statutory responsibilities.

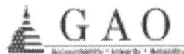

Recommendations to the Agency

- We recommend that the chairman of the Chemical Safety Board
  - develop a plan to address the investigative gap and request the necessary resources from Congress to meet CSB's statutory mandate or seek an amendment to its statutory mandate;
  - consider using the work of other entities, such as government agencies, companies, and contractors (subject to an assessment of the quality of their work) to a greater extent to maximize the board's limited resources; and
  - improve the quality of its accident-screening database by better controlling data entry and periodically sampling accident data to evaluate their consistency and completeness.

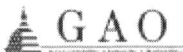

Recommendations to the Agency

- Publish a regulation requiring facilities to report all chemical accidents, as required by law, to better inform the agency of important details about accidents that it may not receive from current sources.
- Consider reinstating the position of chief operating officer, with the delegation of responsibility for establishing performance goals, holding program mangers accountable for meeting those goals, and demonstrating improvement in the agency's ability to meet its statutory mandates over time.
- Use the Strategic Management of Human Capital portion of the President's Management Agenda to provide criteria for developing a comprehensive human capital plan, with input from investigators, that includes specific objectives and performance measures to improve accountability for results and to assist the agency in its goal of improving its human capital and infrastructure.

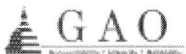

Matters for Congressional Consideration

- Congress may wish to consider amending CSB's organic statute or the Inspector General Act of 1978 to permanently give EPA's Inspector General the authority to serve as the oversight body for the agency.
- As Congress prepares the appropriation of the EPA Inspector General, it may wish to consider providing the Inspector General with appropriations and staff allocations specifically for the audit function of CSB via a direct line in the EPA appropriation.

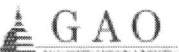

Attachment 1—Federal entities, as defined by the IG Act of 1978

1. Chemical Safety and Hazard Investigation Board*
2. Defense Nuclear Facilities Safety Board*
3. National Transportation Safety Board*
4. Nuclear Waste Technical Review Board*
5. Advisory Council on Historic Preservation
6. African Development Foundation
7. American Battle Monuments Commission
8. Architectural and Transportation Barriers Compliance Board
9. Armed Forces Retirement Home
10. Barry Goldwater Scholarship and Excellence in Education Foundation
11. Christopher Columbus Fellowship Foundation
12. Commission for the Preservation of America's Heritage Abroad
13. Commission of Fine Arts
14. Commission on Civil Rights
15. Committee for Purchase from People Who Are Blind or Severely Disabled

*Has a public safety mission

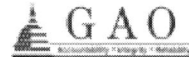

Attachment 1—Federal entities, as defined by the IG Act of 1978

16. Court of Appeals for Veterans Claims
17. Court Services and Offender Supervision Agency for DC
18. Delta Regional Authority
19. Farm Credit System Insurance Corporation
20. Federal Financial Institutions Examination Council
21. Federal Mediation and Conciliation Service
22. Federal Mine Safety and Health Review Commission
23. Federal Retirement Thrift Investment Board
24. Harry S. Truman Scholarship Foundation
25. Inter-American Foundation
26. Institute of American Indian and Alaska Native Culture and Arts Development
27. Institute of Museum and Library Services
28. James Madison Memorial Fellowship Foundation
29. Japan-U.S. Friendship Commission
30. Marine Mammal Commission

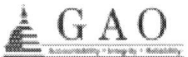

Attachment 1—Federal entities, as defined by the IG Act of 1978

31. Merit Systems Protection Board
32. Millennium Challenge Corporation
33. Morris K. Udall Scholarship and Excellence in National Environmental Policy Foundation
34. National Capital Planning Commission
35. National Commission on Libraries and Information Science
36. National Council on Disability
37. National Mediation Board
38. Neighborhood Reinvestment Corporation
39. Occupational Safety and Health Review Commission
40. Office of Government Ethics
41. Office of Navajo and Hopi Indian Relocation
42. Office of Special Counsel
43. Overseas Private Investment Corporation
44. Presidio Trust
45. Selective Service System

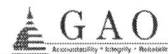

Attachment 1—Federal entities, as defined by the IG Act of 1978

46. Smithsonian Institution/John F. Kennedy Center for the Performing Arts
47. Smithsonian Institution/National Gallery of Art
48. Smithsonian Institution/Woodrow Wilson International Center for Scholars
49. Trade and Development Agency
50. U.S. Holocaust Memorial Museum
51. U.S. Institute of Peace
52. U.S. Interagency Council on Homelessness
53. Vietnam Education Foundation
54. White House Commission on the National Moment of Remembrance

48

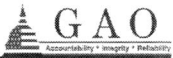

Attachment 2—Types of NTSB Aviation Accident and Incident Investigations

Type of investigations	Number in fiscal year 2006	Description	Travel involved?	Fatalities involved?
Major investigation	7	Investigation of a significant accident that typically involves fatalities, multiple injuries, considerable property damage, or significant public interest. A team of investigators travels to the accident site.	Yes	Yes
Field investigation[a]	196	Investigation of an accident that typically involves a fatality. At least one investigator travels and there is a significant amount of follow-up investigation from the office.	Yes	Typically yes
Limited investigation[a]	550	Investigation of accidents that can involve a fatality but typically do not. Investigators do not travel to the accident site but instead conduct a limited investigation using information collected by Federal Aviation Administration officials, local officials, rescue response units and other persons, and organizations that may have knowledge of the incident.	No	Typically no
Data collection accident investigation	739	Investigations of accidents that do not involve any fatalities, "critical" serious injuries, and other criteria. Investigators do not travel to the accident site but instead collect and analyze information from the office in order to determine the cause.	No	No
Incident investigation[b]	29	Investigation of occurrences that do not involve fatalities. Investigators do not typically travel for these investigations but instead conduct an investigation from the office.	Typically no	No

[a] Includes investigations of public use aircraft.
[b] These occurrences do not meet criteria to be defined as an official accident but are still deemed important enough to investigate.

49

Attachment 3—Types of NTSB Accident Reports

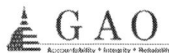

Type	Description
Major accident reports	Reports that provide detailed narrative accounts of the facts, conditions, circumstances, analysis, conclusions, and probable cause of an accident. This type of report is issued for major aviation, railroad, highway, pipeline, and marine accident investigations.
Nonmajor accident reports (or "accident briefs")	Reports that briefly summarize the probable cause of an accident. This type of report is issued for all aviation accidents and for all nonmajor railroad, highway, pipeline, and marine accidents investigated by or for NTSB, for which probable cause is determined.

ENCLOSURE III. COMMENTS FROM CSB

U.S. Chemical Safety and Hazard Investigation Board

2175 K Street, NW • Suite 650 • Washington, DC 20037-1809
Phone: (202) 261-7600 • Fax: (202) 261-7650
www.csb.gov

John S. Bresland
Chairman & CEO

Gary L. Visscher
Board Member

William B. Wark
Board Member

William E. Wright
Board Member

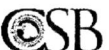

Note: GAO comments supplementing those in the report text appear at the end of this enclosure.

July 11, 2008

John B. Stephenson
Director
Natural Resources and Environment
U.S. Government Accountability Office
441 G Street, N.W.
Washington, DC 20548

Dear Mr. Stephenson:

As requested, we reviewed your draft report, "Chemical Safety Board: Improvements in Management and Oversight are Needed" that your office provided on June 11, 2008. We agree on various points in the draft report, such as the need to expand the investigation program. However, as you are aware, the Chemical Safety and Hazard Investigation Board (CSB) has concerns with many of your conclusions and characterizations. Rather than reiterate our concerns, we will focus our comments on your recommendations.

See comment 1.

Before discussing individual recommendations, however, there is one point that I particularly want to emphasize. The draft report refers to previous Inspector General (IG) recommendations, and leaves the impression, at least, that CSB has not been very responsive to those recommendations. In fact all previous IG recommendations have been closed by the respective IG's who made them.

See comment 2.

Investigative Gap

GAO Recommendation. Develop a plan to address the investigative gap and request the necessary resources from the Congress to meet the CSB's statutory mandate or seek an amendment to its statutory mandate.

See comment 3.

CSB Response. The CSB has not construed the agency's authorizing statute as requiring investigation of *every* chemical accident involving a fatality, serious injury, or substantial property damage, or the potential for such consequences, but understands GAO's concern and recommendation. We also agree that the performance of our mission - to help companies and communities avoid chemical accidents - would be strengthened by investigating and reporting on more of the

United States Accountability Office

U.S. Chemical Safety and Hazard Investigation Board

serious chemical accidents that occur in the United States each year.

See comment 4

In addition to seeking additional investigation resources, we will draft a plan for obtaining information on additional chemical accidents occurring in the United States, and clearly set forth a risk-based approach to accident selection and investigation. We will also work with Congress to clarify the issue of CSB's statutory mandate, as suggested by GAO, including if appropriate, an amendment to the CSB's enabling legislation.

See comment 5

We will examine the work of the National Transportation Safety Board (NTSB) to aid our future plan. However, we note that the GAO's comparison between 6 CSB investigations and 1,521 NTSB aviation investigations in FY 2006 may not be the most fruitful benchmark for future planning. The majority of the NTSB's aviation investigations were non-fatal general aviation incidents, with the NTSB relying heavily on the work of 3,400 FAA regional inspectors to determine the probable cause. Thus, the CSB will also examine the NTSB's statutory authority and work in other modes of transportation. In these other modes, the NTSB

See comment 6

employs a risk based approach to select out priority incidents from all incidents within its jurisdiction.

See comment 7

The purpose of increased resources, the plan, legislative clarification, and other measures discussed below would be to provide greater oversight and analysis of significant chemical incidents in the United States.

Work of Others

GAO Recommendation. Consider using the work of other entities, such as government agencies, companies, and contractors (subject to an assessment of the quality of their work) to maximize the Board's limited resources.

See comment 8

See comment 9

CSB Response. The Board will consider using the work of other entities and contractors to further maximize its limited resources. In our experience, however, there are limits and pitfalls to the use of other entities' work. Based on this experience, we respectfully suggest that the CSB has correctly interpreted its Congressional mandate by independently investigating major accidents and hazards in depth, rather than attempting to serve as a clearinghouse for numerous, disparate, and often superficial reports from other organizations. We discuss some of our initial concerns with GAO's recommendation below.

See comment 10

The Occupational Safety and Health Administration (OSHA) and the Environmental Protection Agency (EPA) frequently conduct inspections at accident sites. However, they have few inspectors focused and specialized on chemical process safety, and these agencies typically do not prepare narrative reports describing what happened and why. Rather, OSHA and EPA may publish citations or notices of regulatory violations, which may or may not relate to the actual causes of the accidents. These lists of violations cannot generally be used to establish and report on the causes of the accidents, as required under the CSB's

Enclosure III. Comments from CSB

**U.S. Chemical Safety and
Hazard Investigation Board**

authorizing statute. Likewise, the investigations conducted by state and local police and fire agencies generally focus on particular inquiries such as the "cause and origin" of a chemical fire, i.e., a determination of the fuel, location, and ignition source. Such narrow determinations fall well short of Congress's stated intentions for the scope of CSB investigations.[1]

See comment 11

In addition, OSHA, EPA, state fire marshals, fire departments, and police clearly have law enforcement and regulatory responsibilities. Investigations by these agencies necessarily focus on rules violations, rather than on the overall adequacy of existing rules, standards, and industry practices. Because of their law enforcement and regulatory duties, many of these agencies are reluctant to share the results of their ongoing investigations with the CSB. In fact, during the CSB's investigation of the BP Texas City disaster, both OSHA and the EPA asserted in correspondence that they would limit the CSB's access to their inspection staff and records, citing in part the possibility of criminal prosecution. Today, more than three years after the BP accident - and more than a year after the CSB completed its landmark 341-page report - issues of criminal responsibility are still being litigated in federal court.

See comment 12

Most companies that experience significant chemical accidents that cause deaths, injuries, or off-site consequences become involved in lengthy litigation proceedings. Even the most enlightened corporations generally produce their own accident investigation reports as part of their litigation defense strategy - not in an effort to inform other companies and the public objectively about underlying causes. Moreover, companies often assert that such reports are protected by legal privilege. Even if the CSB was able to obtain and rely on such reports as a primary source of information, it could undermine the credibility of the CSB's work and lead, in some cases, to incorrectly faulting the efforts of individual workers and third parties, rather than uncovering important systemic causes.

Quality of Accident Data

GAO Recommendation. Improve the quality of [the CSB's] accident screening database by better controlling data entry and periodically sampling accident data to evaluate its consistency and completeness.

CSB Response. We note that the screening database primarily represents a compilation of the earliest reports of accidents – including those from the National Response Center (NRC) and the media – which may contain inherent inaccuracies. Nonetheless the CSB agrees that it should take additional steps to prevent errors from being introduced through incorrect data entry. The CSB will revise its board order on the incident selection process and consider changes to improve data accuracy. We plan to consider such measures as additional written guidance and training for incident screeners; designing an electronic workflow so

---

[1] See S. Rpt. No. 101-228, 1990 U.S.C.C.A.N. 3385, 3617-18 (1989) (stating that, "The Board should take an "all cause" theory . . . . [I]t is expected that the Board will follow many strands of inquiry . . . .")

**U.S. Chemical Safety and
Hazard Investigation Board**

that significant changes to the database require supervisory sign-off; and peri auditing of screening data for quality and completeness. In addition we will review the staffing for the screening program and its overall structure as the (develops its human capital plan. Currently screening is done by junior investigators as collateral duty on a rotating basis. The CSB lacks any staff s dedicated to this task.

Reporting Regulation

GAO Recommendation. Publish a regulation requiring facilities to report all chemi accidents, as required by law, to better inform the agency of important details about accidents that they may not receive from current sources.

See comment 13

CSB Response. The CSB will publish in the Federal Register a Request for Information (RFI) concerning a reporting regulation. The RFI will present various options for rulemaking and seek the views and opinions of our stakeholders on the best path forward. We intend to publish the RFI within t next three months. In addition, the detailed plan to conduct more investigatic will include staffing and resource projections for staff to collect and analyze incident information.

See comment 14

We note that the CSB's position has been that a reporting regulation is not needed for the narrow purpose of notifying the CSB of major accidents warranting the deployment of investigators, which appears to be the sole purpose of the CSB's authority to issue a reporting rule.[2] Given the limited number of investigations that the CSB can conduct, we can and do easily learn what we need to know simply from monitoring the media and reports from the NRC and NTSB.

See comment 15

It is also important to note that the obligation to collect chemical incident dat the broader purposes identified by GAO appears to lie elsewhere in the feder government. For example, Congress funds programs to collect chemical acc: data at both EPA and the Agency for Toxic Substances and Disease Registry OSHA also collects chemical incident information.

Management Accountability and Continuity

GAO Recommendation. Consider reinstating the position of chief operating officer, the delegations of responsibility for establishing performance goals, holding progra managers accountable for meeting those goals, and demonstrating improvement in t agency's ability to meet its statutory mandates over time.

CSB Response. The CSB agrees that it is appropriate to consider establishin; senior executive position to oversee important mission responsibilities. The (

---

[2] See 42 U.S.C. § 7412(r)(6)(C)(iii).

- 4 -

Enclosure III. Comments from CSB

U.S. Chemical Safety and
Hazard Investigation Board

See comment 16.

will give serious consideration to the establishment of such a position as part of its development of a strategic human capital plan.

We note that GAO presented no evidence of a problem by not having a Chief Operating Officer (COO); rather they simply assert the CSB has "longstanding, serious, and intractable management problems." This is in stark contrast to the reality that the CSB's highest impact products (BP Texas City, Combustible Dust Study, CTA, Baker Panel, and the Safety Video Program) are from the post-2004 era when there was no COO. The GAO overlooks the fact that during the five years from 1998 to 2002, the CSB completed a total of 12 investigations but then went on to complete 35 investigations from 2003 to 2008 – a near tripling of productivity on a flat budget.

It is also important to note that the CSB was without a Chairperson from August 2, 2007 to March 17, 2008, virtually the entire duration of the GAO's review. Consistent with its protocols, the Board delegated one Member interim executive and administrative authority to ensure orderly continuation of functions and duties, and there were no accountability or continuity issues identified during this period. Therefore, as the Board has evolved, the concern that the "CSB may not be able to ensure continuity of performance and accountability when Board Members and Chairs leave the agency," should be considered in the context of recent events which suggest otherwise.

Human Capital Issues

GAO Recommendation. Use the Strategic Management of Human Capital portion of the President's Management Agenda as criteria for developing a comprehensive human capital plan, with input from investigators that includes specific objectives and performance measures to improve accountability for results and to assist the agency in its goal of improving its human capital and infrastructure.

CSB Response. The CSB agrees to use the Strategic Management of Human Capital portion of the President's Management Agenda (PMA) as a guide for developing a comprehensive human capital plan.[3] The CSB will also continue to work with the Office of Personnel Management's (OPM) Small Agencies Human Capital Leadership and Merit System Accountability Office to develop the human capital plan. In addition, as recommended by OPM, the CSB will use the "Human Capital Report and Plan for the CSB's Office of Investigations" developed by the CSB human capital team in October of 2005 to help guide development of the comprehensive human capital plan. Developing the plan will be included in the CSB's FY 2009 action plan.

---

[3] OPM indicated to the CSB that it is not a scored agency under the PMA and therefore not required to go to the depth a scored agency must. However, the CSB will develop the human capital plan using the PMA as a guide.

- 5 -

U.S. Chemical Safety and Hazard Investigation Board

Matters for Congressional Consideration

Finally, GAO's draft report raised two specific matters for Congressional consideration concerning oversight of the CSB. The CSB supports oversight and agrees that the CSB authorizing legislation or the IG Act of 1978 are the proper places to address CSB oversight. However, the CSB has concerns with the GAO's specific suggestions for Congressional consideration.

GAO Suggestion. Congress may wish to consider amending the CSB's authorizing statute or the Inspector General Act of 1978 to permanently give the EPA's Inspector General the authority to serve as the oversight body for the agency.

See comment 17

CSB Comment. The CSB respectfully disagrees with the GAO's suggestion that the EPA IG is the best, if not only, approach to provide permanent oversight for the CSB. While the EPA IG is one option for oversight of the CSB, other Offices of Inspector General are also available, some of which may be more appropriate for the role.

See comment 18

There are other alternatives as well. For example, the CSB is modeled on the NTSB. The NTSB, a much larger agency than the CSB, has never had and does not have its own Inspector General. Rather, GAO and the Department of Transportation Inspector General (DOTIG) share oversight responsibilities. GAO is responsible for broad oversight of the NTSB.[4] DOTIG is limited "to review *only* the financial management, property management, and business operations of the National Transportation Safety Board." (Emphasis added.)[5] DOTIG actually contracts this function to a third party which it oversees, so the connection between DOTIG and the NTSB is extremely limited.

See comment 19

This model has been established in recognition of the fact that the NTSB issues recommendations to the Department of Transportation, similar to the manner in which the CSB issues recommendations to the EPA. Indeed, Congress has *consistently* and specifically *rejected* the assignment of DOTIG to serve as the Inspector General of the NTSB.[6] The relevant legislative history explains that the limited nature of the DOTIG's authority was to "ensure that Inspector General oversight does not undermine the independence of the NTSB."[7]

See comment 20

Another alternative is a small in-house Inspector General office. Such a model already exists for about 30 medium-size agencies, such as the Consumer Product Safety Commission, which are not large enough to have presidentially appointed

---

[4] See Pub. L. No. 109-443, 120 Stat. 3297, 3299, § 5(a) (2006) (codified at 49 U.S.C.A. § 1138).
[5] 49 U.S.C. § 1137(a).
[6] The CSB has conducted numerous discussions with NTSB officials in order to understand why the DOTIG role as the NTSB IG was rejected. NTSB officials have consistently explained to us that this was to prevent the appearance or the occurrence of conflicts with DOT officials to whom the NTSB makes recommendations.
[7] H.R. Rep. No. 106-335 at 9 (2000) and S. Rep. 106-386 at 9 (2000).

Enclosure III. Comments from CSB

See comment 21.

U.S. Chemical Safety and Hazard Investigation Board

IG's. Such an arrangement would appear to be less costly and more beneficial in the long term than what GAO has suggested.

GAO Suggestion. As Congress prepares the appropriation of the EPA Inspector General it may wish to consider providing the Inspector General with appropriations and staff allocations specifically for the audit function of CSB via a direct line in the budget.

CSB Comment. The CSB is concerned that GAO did not adequately consider different oversight options for the CSB. While we agree that oversight of every federal agency is appropriate and can be beneficial, it should be tailored to the size of the agency. In that regard I note that the CSB currently obtains its financial and information security audits for about $60,000 a year.

* * *

Thank you for the opportunity to comment on your draft report.

Sincerely,

John S. Bresland
Chairman & CEO

The following are GAO's comments to the U.S. Chemical Safety and Hazard Investigation Board's letter dated August 9, 2008.

GAO Evaluation

1. We believe this briefing fairly and factually identifies continuing problems with CSB's governance, management, and oversight that have continued since we first reported on CSB, in fiscal year 2000.[1] We conducted this performance audit in accordance with generally accepted government auditing standards. Those standards require that we plan and perform the audit to obtain sufficient, appropriate evidence to provide a reasonable basis for our findings and conclusions based on our audit objectives. We believe that the

---

[1] GAO, *Chemical Safety Board: Improved Policies and Additional Oversight Are Needed* (GAO/RCED-00-192, July 11, 2000).

evidence obtained provides a reasonable basis for our findings and conclusions based on our audit objectives.

2. While the inspectors general closed these recommendations, their decision was often based on CSB's commitment to take future actions and the IG's reserving the right to reopen recommendations. As stated in the briefing, our analysis shows that CSB has not fully responded to key recommendations related to (1) investigating more accidents that meet statutory requirements triggering C SB's responsibility to investigate, (2) improving the quality of its accident data, (3) resolving human capital problems, and (4) ensuring accountability and continuity of management.

3. The 1990 Clean Air Act Amendments establishing CSB contained the following mandates:

- "The Board shall investigate (or cause to be investigated)... *any* accidental release resulting in a fatality, serious injury or substantial property damage"[2] (emphasis added).
- "*In no event shall the Board forgo* an investigation where an accidental release causes a fatality or serious injury among the general public, or had [sic] *the potential* to cause substantial property damage or a number of deaths or injuries among the general public"[3] (emphasis added).

    As noted in our briefing slides, this language clearly identifies the accidental releases CSB is required to investigate; investigations are required for all accidental releases that result, or have the potential to result, in a fatality, serious injury, or substantial property damage.

4. While CSB reports that it will seek additional investigation resources and "will draft a plan for obtaining information on additional chemical accidents occurring in the United States, and clearly set forth a risk-based approach to accident selection and investigation," it does not commit to meet C SB's statutory mandate or commit to investigating more than six accidents per year. However, CSB reported that the agency would work with Congress to clarify the issue of its statutory

---

[2] 42 U.S.C. § 7412(r)(6)(C)(i).

mandate and, if appropriate, seek an amendment to its authorizing statute.

Also see comment 3.

5. A more useful benchmark for comparison between CSB and NTSB is to examine their appropriations and accident investigations. As noted on slide 15, while NTSB's budget is 8 times CSB's budget, NTSB investigated 250 times as many accidents. In addition, while CSB notes that the majority of NTSB's accident investigations were nonfatal, the majority of accidents CSB screened were also nonfatal, as stated on slide 14.

CSB also notes that NTSB relies "heavily on the work of FAA." CSB could similarly rely more on the work of EPA and OSHA and already has cooperative agreements in place with these agencies to share information on accidents. The agency currently has memorandums of understanding (MOU) with both EPA and OSHA with the stated purpose of establishing "policy and general procedures for cooperation and coordination between the two Agencies to minimize duplication of activities." Moreover, the MOUs state the two agencies will "coordinate incident notification, data and information exchange, training, technical and professional assistance." The MOU with EPA further states that "in certain instances, the CSB may decide not to send an investigation team to the site of a chemical incident. Rather, CSB may collect incident information from EPA or other on-site agencies compiled in the course of their own actions." Similar language appears in the MOU with OSHA.

6. In our view, this approach would not be consistent with CSB's own authorizing legislation. NTSB's authorizing legislation gives it broad discretion in determining which accidents in the nonaviation transportation modes to investigate. For example, NTSB "shall investigate or have investigated... a highway accident, including a railroad grade crossing accident, the Board selects in cooperation with a State"4 (emphasis added). In addition, NTSB's authorizing legislation requires investigations of "any other accident related to the transportation of individuals or property when the Board decides" that

---

[3] 42 U.S.C. § 7412(r)(6)(E).
[4] 49 U.S.C. § 1131(a)(1)(B).

certain circumstances are present (emphasis added).5 CSB's authorizing statute, on the other hand, does not contain any similar language providing discretion for CSB to determine which accidental releases to investigate.

CSB's statutory authority is more comparable to the language that governs NTSB's investigations of civil aviation, railroad, and pipeline accidents. NTSB is required to investigate railroad accidents with a fatality or substantial property, railroad accidents that involve a passenger train, and pipeline accidents with fatalities, substantial property damage, or significant injury to the environment.6 Like CSB, NTSB is required to investigate these types of accidents; it does not have the discretion to choose which to investigate.

Also see comment 3 and 4.

7. Our recommendation is to develop a plan to address the investigative gap and request the necessary resources from Congress to meet CSB's statutory mandate or seek an amendment to its statutory mandate.

Also see comment 3 and 6.

8. GAO agrees that there are limitations in using the work of others. As CSB examines NTSB's work, it may find that there are lessons to be learned about how to minimize the limitations in using the work of others. While NTSB uses its authority to solicit the investigative work performed by others when resources or other considerations prevent it from deploying to accident sites, in all cases, overall investigative control—including determination of probable cause—rests with NTSB. As we reported in 2007, outside experts provide critical assistance to NTSB investigators. During the course of an investigation, NTSB supplements its investigative staff through the use of "parties" and outside contractors when it needs additional support for fact finding or technical analysis. "Party" participants include individuals, agencies, companies, and associations that can provide technical expertise relevant to a specific accident during the fact-finding phase. While the party process may provide technical information that is important for determining the cause of an accident,

---

[5] 49 U.S.C. § 1131(a)(1)(F).
[6] 42 U.S.C. § 1131(a)(1).

it presents inherent conflicts of interest for entities that are both parties in an investigation and potential defendants in related litigation. For example, in a commercial aviation accident, the principal defendants in litigation for damages are likely to be the airline and aircraft manufacturer, who may face liability for dozens of deaths—both entities that are likely working with NTSB as parties to the investigation. Despite such challenges, the party system appears to be working well; for example, RAND Corporation found that the party system works well in that it allows NTSB to leverage its resources to provide critical safety information in regard to the accident under investigation. In addition, NTSB officials told us that the system is an efficient way of gathering and sharing information about the accident with investigators and other parties. Also, having multiple parties on an investigation offsets concerns of conflict of interest and impartiality.

In addition, according to NTSB officials, the agency makes a distinction between fact gathering and analysis. Parties are permitted to gather facts (evidence) for NTSB, but they are not permitted to engage in the analysis of that evidence.

9. As noted above, CSB's authorizing statute requires investigations of all accidental releases that cause, or have the potential to cause, a fatality, serious injury, or substantial property damage. CSB's authorizing statute does not specify, that investigations should be limited to those accidental releases that are "major." In addition, CSB's authorizing statute grants CSB discretion to "utilize the expertise and experience of other agencies."[7]

    Also see comment 3.

10. CSB could use information available from other entities, including OSHA and EPA, to conduct its own independent analysis of accidents, although in some cases, CSB may need to supplement information provided by other entities through follow-up calls, sending investigators to the scene of the accident, or other means.

    Also see comment 8.

---

[7] 42 U.S.C. § 7412(r)(6)(D).

11. When CSB examines the work of NTSB, the agency could review how NTSB obtains information from other public entities pertaining to ongoing investigations.

    Also, see comments 5 and 8.

12. An examination of NTSB's work may provide information about how NTSB uses its party process to minimize the limitations in using the work of others.

    Also see comments 8 and 11.

13. We recognize that obtaining the views and opinions of CSB's stakeholders could provide valuable information regarding the preparation of a reporting regulation. However, the request for information does not in itself provide assurance that CSB will follow through and issue a regulation as required by CSB's authorizing statute. Specifically, the statute provides that the board "shall... establish by regulation requirements binding on persons for reporting accidental releases into the ambient air subject to the Board's investigatory jurisdiction."[8] CSB's comments concerning the need for such a regulation are not relevant because CSB is legally required to promulgate a regulation. In addition, we disagree with CSB about the regulation's usefulness. A reporting regulation would allow CSB to obtain more accurate, complete information to meet its statutory mandate.

14. As we note in our briefing, information reported by facilities would be a better source than CSB's current practice of relying mostly on information from the media, which CSB officials acknowledge is often inaccurate or incomplete. Our analysis of C SB's accident data showed that in fiscal year 2007, CSB received 66 percent of its chemical accident notifications exclusively from the news media. In addition, CSB's accident database is not just for selection of accidents to investigate, it is also used to report to Congress and serves as a historical record of information on chemical accidents that could be used to identify trends and patterns in chemical accidents and prevent future accidents.

See also comment 13.

15. The Department of Homeland Security Inspector General (DHS IG) reported in 2004 that the lack of comprehensive and timely reporting on chemical accidents in general is a problem the CSB is both positioned and required to address.[9] Citing a 2002 CSB report on reactive hazards,[10] the DHS IG reported that "CSB searched 40 public and private databases and reported that its findings were limited because existing sources of incident data are inadequate to identify the number, severity, frequency, and causes of reactive incidents. CSB's analysis included chemical accident data at EPA and OSHA.

Also see comments 13 and 14.

16. We introduced the recommendation for reinstating a permanent COO as one way CSB could begin addressing the management and accountability problems that we have presented in this briefing. As stated in the briefing, the difficulties that CSB has experienced in meeting its mission are largely the result of inadequate management accountability for addressing long-standing problems. If CSB officials recognize these long-standing problems and agree that they need to be addressed, then reinstating a permanent COO could help provide the continuity of management needed to bring about this change. In addition, former Chairman Carolyn W. Merritt testified in July 2007 that CSB

> "would benefit...if Congress... provided for a vice chairman to assure the orderly transition during times when the chair is vacant. Periodic vacancies in the chair, and the resulting absence of executive authority, pose a significant risk to the success of the agency. Under the existing structure, CSB board members cannot serve beyond the expiration of their five-year terms, and thus vacancies in the chair and other board seats are all but inevitable."[11]

---

[8] 42 U.S.C. § 7412(r)(6)(C)(iii).
[9] Department of Homeland Security Office of Inspector General, *A Report on the Continuing Development of the U.S. Chemical Safety and Hazard Investigation Board,* OIG-04-04 (Jan. 7, 2004).
[10] U.S. Chemical Safety and Hazard Investigation Board, *Improving Reactive Hazard Management*, Sept. 17, 2002.
[11] Testimony of Carolyn W. Merritt, Chairman and Chief Executive Officer, U.S. Chemical Safety and Hazard Investigation Board before the U.S. Senate Committee on Environment

17. While we recognize that alternatives exist for providing CSB with management oversight, after reviewing various oversight options, we continue to believe that the EPA IG has several advantages, provides the best option for oversight, and the oversight authority should be made permanent. The EPA IG has expertise involving the chemical management issues that the Board is charged with investigating, has gained knowledge of CSB's operations and activities in providing the Board with oversight over the past several years, and, like other IGs, has the requisite independence provided by the IG Act of 1978 necessary for reviewing and making recommendations to address longstanding problems in the Board's management performance.

18. We recognize that Congress provided for a division of responsibility between the Department of Transportation (DoT) IG and GAO regarding the oversight of NTSB. However, GAO has largely devoted its efforts to program evaluations and policy analyses that look at programs and functions across government and with a longer-term perspective. On the other hand, IGs have been on the front line of combating fraud, waste, and abuse within their respective agencies, and their work has generally concentrated on specific program-related issues of immediate concern with more of their resources going into uncovering inappropriate activities and expenditures through an emphasis on investigations. IGs play a critical role in identifying mismanagement of scarce taxpayer dollars and could provide, based on the results of our evaluation, a valuable service for the CSB. Moreover, as we have stated in the past, we believe that all significant federal programs and entities should be subject to oversight by independent IGs.

    See comment 17.

19. In response to CSB's point that Congress has "consistently and specifically rejected" assigning the DoT IG to serve as IG of the NTSB, we note that the DoT IG's assignment to and GAO annual audit requirements of the NTSB are recent actions—the DoT IG was

---

and Public Works, Subcommittee on Transportation Safety, Infrastructure Security, and Water Quality, July 10, 2007.

assigned to NTSB in 2000 and GAO assigned in late 2006. As stated in the briefing, we believe that all significant federal programs and entities should be subject to oversight by IGs who can provide sound, independent audits of all significant federal operations and activities. While we recognize that the Congress took specific actions it felt appropriate to ensure the independence of NTSB, we note that Congress has not taken such action with respect to CSB. Furthermore, IGs are independent from the agency they audit and investigate, and we believe the EPA IG has the requisite independence from CSB.

See comment 17 and 18.

20. As stated in the briefing, CSB's history of management problems warrants a level of independent oversight that may be difficult to achieve by an internal audit function. In addition, the limited staffing that would reasonably be allocated to this function at an agency of this size would lack the varied expertise needed to address these problems.

21. As stated in the briefing, we believe that all significant federal programs and entities should be subject to oversight by IGs who can provide sound, independent audits of all significant federal operations and activities. Given the management problems that our audit revealed, the need for independent IG oversight is especially pressing. We also note that these management problems would not be addressed by financial or information security audits.

See comment 17, 19 and 20.

INDEX

A

accident prevention, 26
accidents, vii, viii, ix, 11, 12, 13, 15, 16, 17, 19, 20, 21, 26, 27, 28, 29, 33, 34, 37, 38, 72, 73, 74, 75, 76, 77
accountability, vii, 12, 15, 23, 27, 30, 72, 77
accuracy, 21
alternative, 12, 27
alternatives, 78
ambient air, 76
assessment, 29
assignment, 26, 78
auditing, 13, 38, 71
authority, viii, 12, 16, 20, 23, 31, 34, 74, 77, 78

B

binding, 76
board members, 23, 24, 77

C

chain of command, 23
Clean Air Act, 11, 33, 72
compensation, 23
compliance, 12
conflict, 75
conflict of interest, 75
Congress, vii, 11, 12, 15, 19, 20, 21, 25, 26, 29, 31, 33, 72, 74, 76, 77, 78
continuity, vii, 15, 23, 24, 26, 72, 77
control, 12, 74

D

database, 13, 21, 29, 33, 37, 38, 76
deaths, 34, 72, 75
decisions, 27
defendants, 75
Department of Homeland Security, 12, 77
division, 78
draft, 33, 72
duplication, 73
duration, 25

E

employees, 22, 26
engagement, 37
environment, 74

Environmental Protection Agency, 12
EPA, viii, 12, 17, 21, 26, 28, 31, 34, 73, 75, 77, 78, 79
expenditures, 78
expertise, ix, 17, 25, 34, 74, 75, 78, 79

F

FEMA, 12, 22, 23
fraud, 78
funding, vii, 15
funds, 23

G

goals, 22, 23, 29
governance, vii, 12, 15, 71
government, 13, 29, 38, 71, 78
grants, 75
guidance, 37

H

hazardous substances, 11
hazards, 77
hiring, 22
House, 12, 36
human capital, vii, 12, 15, 19, 22, 27, 30, 33, 37, 72
human resources, 22

I

independence, viii, 17, 21, 25, 26, 34, 78, 79
industry, 22
information exchange, 73
infrastructure, 30
injuries, 21, 27, 28, 34, 37, 72
inspectors, viii, 17, 26, 34, 72

intervention, 23

J

jobs, 23
jurisdiction, 76

L

language, 34, 72, 73, 74
legislation, 73
likelihood, 11
litigation, 75

M

management, vii, ix, 12, 15, 17, 19, 22, 23, 24, 25, 27, 34, 35, 37, 71, 72, 77, 78, 79
mandates, 27, 29, 72
manufacturer, 75
measures, 11, 22, 30
media, 21, 27, 76

N

narratives, 37
newspapers, 21

O

Office of Management and Budget, 20, 26
organizations, 20, 27
oversight, vii, viii, 12, 15, 16, 25, 26, 31, 34, 35, 37, 71, 78, 79

P

planning, 22
private sector, 23
program, 20, 22, 23, 26, 29, 34, 35, 37, 78
public safety, 12

Q

quality control, 13, 21, 38

R

regulation, viii, 16, 21, 27, 29, 76
regulations, 11, 21, 37
relationship, 25, 26
reliability, 37
resources, vii, 15, 19, 20, 22, 26, 27, 28, 29, 33, 72, 74, 78
retention, 22
risk, ix, 17, 26, 33, 34, 72, 77

S

safety, 11, 12, 23, 75
sampling, 29
security, 35, 79
Senate, 12, 35, 77
severity, 77
sharing, 75
skills, 24
staffing, 25, 79
stakeholders, viii, 16, 76
standards, 13, 28, 38, 71
statutes, 37

T

television, 21
time, 12, 21, 22, 23, 24, 29
training, 73
transition, 77
transportation, 73

U

United States, 12, 33, 35, 72

V

vacancies, 77
variables, 37

W

warrants, 25, 79